I0116603

# Glow UP and Sparkle

## A Self-Love Book for Women

by

## R. G. Collins, Ed.D

Glow Up and Sparkle

A Self Love Book for Women

Published by Dr. Rhonda G. Collins

COPYRIGHT ©2021 DR. RHONDA G. COLLINS.
All rights reserved.

No part of this book may be reproduced in any form or by any mechanical means, including information storage and retrieval systems without permission in writing from the publisher/author, except by a
reviewer who may quote passages in a review.

All images, logos, quotes, and trademarks included in this book are subject to use according to trademark and copyright laws of the UnitedStates of America.

COLLINS, G. RHONDA DR. Author GLOW UP AND SPARKLE

A SELF LOVE BOOK FOR WOMENDR. RHONDA G. COLLINS

ISBN : 978-1-7365767-6-2

All rights reserved by DR. RHONDA G. COLLINS. The book is printed in the United States of America.

## Acknowledgements

This book is dedicated to all of the young women at heart who love themselves, who are learning to love themselves, and who love life.

# Love Yourself First

# Table of Contents

# GLOW UP TO

# TO SELF LOVE

## INTRODUCTION

Throughout my thirty plus year career in the education profession, I have enjoyed counseling children and adolescents. My training and education have allowed me to assist children in a variety of areas including academic, emotional, behavioral, adjustment, family, and social concerns.

My counseling sessions were designed to work with children and adolescents in groups or individually, depending on the situation. I've helped students make the best decisions for their future.

I also worked with parents of each child I've counseled to help them understand what is best for their child and to learn ways to help their child deal with multiple self-awareness concerns.

One of my greatest joys involved bi-weekly meetings with the female groups I've advised and facilitated. We have worked on self-esteem, self-confidence, self-awareness, cyber bullying and anti- bullying tactics, table manners and etiquette, college and career awareness to name a few.

I would sometimes see young women who were not aware of self-love and were afraid to put their best interests before that of others. I absolutely love helping young women learn to love themselves.

This love has inspired me to write this book, Glow Up and Glitter and its companion, the journal with Glow Up and Sparkle. I could only hope that my love for their success and discovery of self-love can be manifested into their being.

This book was created and designed with the you in mind. The Glow Up and Sparkle Journal is a perfect companion to the book. When this pair is combined, they provide an opportunity for personal growth and development, as well as change for your mind-set in the areas of self-esteem, self-confidence, and self-awareness.

While completing the journal entries, note the feelings and emotions you are feeling at the time.

When you reach the final entry of the journal and the final page of the book, your perception of self should be impacted. The final desire is for you to Love Yourself First.

If you love yourself first, you will not lose yourself while trying to pleas others.  Be happy with yourself. Know who you are.

Don't allow others to dictate your journey and who you are as a person.

The cover for the book and the title of the book emphasizes how we are always growing into the people that we want to be. Your journey should look somewhat like the journey of a butterfly.  Like a butterfly, we grow from a caterpillar (small child), crawling around and learning from our environment. Then we find go a safe warm place where we cocoon. Here we are truly unable to see what is around us, inside of us, and in front of us because there may be blinders or a thick skin that is preventing us from seeing our magnificent beauty. Often times, we don't realize that we are changing and evolving. We are blooming and growing a hundred times our previous size and into the graceful, confident, and beautiful butterfly that we had inside of us all along.

I know you are excited to take this journey of growth and development. This book and journal will help you take flight along the way.

I have my experience as a counselor and as a woman growing into life and life growing into me prepared me to write this self-help book for you and me.

The way women see ourselves is very important. We dim our light so that someone else's light can shine. Your light can be shine so brightly. Allow it to glow and sparkle without shame, guilt, fear, or regret. Fear sometimes holds back our own glow up.

When you see where you are, you will be able to look back over time to see the progress you have made.

The way we see ourselves is a reflection of how we feel about our self. The current feeling or perception of self during the beginning of this book may change by the time you reach the end of this book and the journal. That is the goal. Enjoy your journey.

# WHAT IS HER GLOW-CONFIDENCE?

Over the years, I have grown to love myself more and more each day. At one point in my life, I had very little self-confidence. I put a lot of other people's feelings before my own. I dimmed my life to allow other's light to shine.  My confidence was very low.  I think my mother saw something in me that I could not see.  I would tell her stories about situations and people I in my life. I sometimes thought other people were smarter or had a better life. As time went on, I realized a lot of people either live a false life or made their life appear as if it was wonderful but it wasn't.

When considering self-confidence, we think of an attitude about your abilities and capabilities. It implies that you embrace and trust yourself and that you are in command of your life. You know your strengths and weaknesses well and you have a positive view of self. You set realistic goals and expectations, communicates assertively, and can handle criticism.

On the other hand, low self-confidence can make you feel self-doubtful, passive or submissive, or have a hard time trusting others. You may feel inferior, unloved, or sensitive to criticism. Feeling confident can depend on the situation. For example, you may feel very confident in some areas, such as academics, but not be confident in others, such as relationships.

Having high or low self-confidence is often dependent on your expectations, not your real skills. Perceptions are the way you think about yourself and these thoughts can be wrong.

Low self-confidence can be due to different experiences, such as growing up in a critical and unsupported environment, separating from your friends or family for the first time, judging yourself too harshly, or having a fear of failure. People with low self-confidence often have thinking errors.

Self-confidence is knowing that you can trust your own judgments and skills, and that you respect and feel deserving of yourself, despite any flaws or what others can think of you.

Self-efficacy and self-esteem are often confused with self-confidence, but they are not the same thing.

We acquire a sense of self-efficacy when we see ourselves (and others like us) mastering skills and achieving goals. This gives us hope that if we learn and work hard in a specific field, we can succeed. It is this kind of trust that leads people to accept difficult challenges and to move on in the face of setbacks.

Self-esteem is a more general sense that we can cope with what happens in our lives and that we have the right to be happy.

Furthermore, self-esteem comes in part from the feeling that the people around us approve of us. We may or may not be able to control this. If we are subjected to a lot of criticism or disapproval from others, our self-esteem may suffer unless we have additional help.

Confidence is what turns thoughts into actions. Without it we repress ourselves or hold ourselves back from achieving. We need it to get into action and define self-confidence as a belief as well as a feeling.

Confidence is also a belief that we can achieve a successful result through our actions. In other words, when we are sure that we believe that we are good enough, we believe that we have value to offer, and those beliefs are what lead us to take action. For example, to apply for a job, to ask for that promotion or to approach your boss for a raise.

Trust is also something we feel in our body. It may be difficult to pin down, but it is a feeling we have inside. For some, it could be a feeling of enthusiasm or passion or a feeling of calm or serenity. Confidence is a feeling that we experience within ourselves.

So, to understand trust, we have to look at both the mind and the body for answers.

Complete the following entry from the Glow Up and Sparkle journal:

Draw a picture of yourself or place a picture of yourself on this page.

This will allow you to look at yourself at the beginning of your journey to see how you look, what feelings you may have about your life at the time, and also what you think of yourself. How much do you love yourself on a scale of 1 to 10?

# Why is Glow Confidence So Important?

There has long been a common belief among professional women that if you work hard, that will be enough to get you ahead. I want to break this myth. The truth is, it is NOT really enough to be competent and perform well at your job.

To be competitive, you must be competent and optimistic. You need both!

But many women make the mistake of concentrating solely on proving themselves through performance. They overlook other acts that are needed to boost their personal brand and visibility within an organization.

To boost your image and gain exposure, you need to be able to step out of your comfort zone and build relationships with key decision makers. You need to be able to express your opinions and speak in meetings, make presentations, and find ways to showcase your accomplishments. You must be authentic and earn the trust of others. And here's the thing: all of these things require you to have confidence in yourself.

I know this first-hand because I have dealt with a very strong internal bully myself and have had to overcome a lack of self-confidence and self-esteem in order to step up to my full potential. I used to be so afraid of saying the wrong thing and embarrassing myself that I would literally keep quiet during team meetings. "You are too young to be in this position," my inner bully would say, or "If you speak up, people will find out that you are a liar and not confident." So, I'd just sit there, not contributing any thoughts or opinions.

And of course, this was a self-fulfilling prophecy. The more I kept quiet, the more people probably thought I had nothing to add of value. So, my greatest fear manifested itself! But it wasn't because I said anything inappropriate; instead, my Inner Bully told me that I wasn't good enough.

Not feeling good enough is the biggest barrier to following our dreams, making changes in our lives, and bringing our ideas to the world. With this lack of self-confidence, we hold back and get stuck in our comfort zone, eventually leading to feelings of inadequacy, low self-esteem, and a lack of drive and motivation.

Complete the following entry from the Glow Up and Sparkle journal:

I Love myself because....

# WHY HER GLOW-CONFIDENCE MATTERS

While self-confidence is important in almost every aspect of our lives, many people struggle to find it. Unfortunately, this can be a vicious cycle - people who lack self-confidence are less likely to achieve the success that could give them more confidence.

For example, you may not want to endorse a project submitted by someone who is visibly nervous, clumsy, or constantly apologizing. On the other hand, someone who speaks clearly, holds their head up, answers questions confidently, and readily admit when they don't know something, can persuade you.

Confident people inspire trust in others: your audience, your coworkers, your bosses, your customers, and your friends. And earning the trust of others is one of the key ways to be successful. I'll show you how to do it in the parts below.

## HOW TO APPEAR MORE CONFIDENT TO OTHERS

You can show self-confidence in many ways: in your behavior, your body language, and what you say and how you say it.

Self-confidence can be improved by projecting a positive picture to others. It's not just a case of "faking it." Others are more likely to react positively if you project trust. This positive reinforcement will make you believe in yourself.

**Body language**

Here are some general tips to help you look and feel more confident.

Take an open posture. Place your hands at your sides and sit or stand up straight. Standing with your hands on your hips communicates your desire to be in command. Make sure you're not hunched over! Do not cross arms.

Keep your head straight and upright. Maintain a close relationship between your upper arms and your body. I will talk more about this later.

I will talk more about body language later.

Complete the following entry from the Glow Up and Sparkle journal:

I feel beautiful in my own skin and with my body because...

## Face to face communication

People with low self-confidence often have a hard time making a good first impression, whether they're meeting someone, heading to a meeting, or giving a presentation. You may be shy or unsure of yourself, but you can take immediate action to make yourself appear more confident.

It is important to interact with people, so keep eye contact as you speak. This shows that you are interested in what they are saying and that you are actively participating in the conversation. But be aware of cultural considerations when it comes to body language and communication.

Don't fidget or look away as you continue the conversation, as this can make you appear distracted or anxious.

If shaking hands is the standard greeting at your place of business, or personal encounters, be firm. However, don't be too firm and avoid being too direct. Reaching for the other person's wrist or shoulder with your free hand is often considered a way to establish dominance, and is not recommended for a first meeting. Avoid making the encounter uncomfortable or worse, painful.

Complete the following entry from the Glow Up and Sparkle journal:

When I walk in a crowded room, I feel...


# MEETING SHORT-TERM CHALLENGES TO YOUR

# RADIANT SELF-CONFIDENCE

Even the most confident person can sometimes find themselves doubting their abilities. For example, you may have a talent for coming up with great ideas or solutions, but find it difficult to make her voice heard. You may suddenly have to work from home for a long period of time and feel lost or isolated without the company of your colleagues or friends.

To solve short-term morale drops, first try to figure out what's causing the problem.

If you're having trouble keeping your faith because of stuff you think you can't do, it's time to brush up on your skills. To define your strengths and weaknesses, write on a sheet of paper a list that includes both. Then come up with an action plan to work on the areas where you are not as strong.

The attitudes or behavior of other people can contribute to your lack of confidence. If you are being harassed, if you are subject to micro-injuries, or if you feel that people are making unfair assumptions about you, let the person know how you feel about their behavior. Report this behavior, if it occurs in the work place or school setting.

Practice assertiveness to create a sense that you have rights and needs as an individual, and make sure others understand and respect your personal limits. This will help you develop the psychological security you need to build self-confidence.

# How do you earn and maintain glow-confidence?

Short-term action can help with immediate or acute trust issues, but long-term confidence building necessitates more fundamental action. This may mean making lifestyle changes and making solid plans for the future.

## Building trust habits

Aim to cultivate positive habits (and break bad ones!) in order to develop a healthy sense of self-worth and the trust that comes with it.

Take control of your physical and emotional health by exercising on a daily basis. Make sure you get enough rest and eat a balanced diet. Failure to do so can make you feel bad about yourself.

Working on your personal brand can also have a positive impact on your self-confidence. If you can project a positive image of your authentic self, you are likely to start receiving positive feedback that is so important to your self-confidence.

## Review of past achievements

Your self-confidence can increase when you can say, "I can do this, and here's the evidence." As part of your personal SWOT (strengths, weaknesses, opportunities, and threats) analysis, you will have identified the things you are good at, based on your past accomplishments.

List the 10 things you are most proud of in an "achievement log." Perhaps you rose to the top on an important test or exam, played a key role in an important team or project, or did something that made a positive difference in someone else's life.

Examine your achievements and use them to make optimistic affirmations about your abilities. If you have a tendency to undermine your own self-confidence with negative self-talk, these affirmations can be especially effective. I will discuss affirmations in more detail later.

## Set goals that will help your confidence glow.

Setting and achieving goals is an important aspect of self-confidence growth. The process of setting goals and determining how good you are is known as goal setting.

Your own SWOT review will help you set goals. Set goals that make the most of your strengths, minimize your weaknesses, seize your opportunities, and mitigate the threats you face.

Determine the first move for each of the key goals you want to accomplish after you've defined them. Make sure it's a short step. It shouldn't take more than an hour to finish.

If you start to have questions when setting goals, write them down and challenge them calmly and rationally. It's better if they seem less serious when questioned. However, if they are based on real risks, be sure to set additional goals to manage them appropriately.

Breaking down big goals into smaller steps in this way makes them seem much more achievable. It also allows you to track your progress and reflect on how far you've come so far.

# WHY WOMEN HAVE A DULL

# SELF ESTEEM

Self-esteem is your opinion of yourself. People who have a good sense of self-worth are proud of themselves and their accomplishments. Although everyone loses trust from time to time, people with low self-esteem are generally unhappy or disappointed with themselves. This can be remedied, but it takes care and daily practice to boost self-esteem.

When I look in the mirror and I see something beautiful, I love what I see. I feel beautiful in my own skin and with my body.

Sometimes we are concerned about people viewing us in a certain way. We worry about what others think of us. We should not worry about what others says or think about us because this can make us feel worthless. We have to improve our self-esteem. We are our own experts when it comes to self. There is no other person in this world who is more aware of who we are other than self.

Having good self-esteem is essential to be able to enjoy a fuller and more satisfying life, in addition to allowing us to live it as we want. Often, the lack of self-esteem can enable us to be manipulated by stronger people or not live the life we want due to lack of self-love.

## Types of Self-Esteem

In a general way, one can speak of two types of self-esteem, although they are not whole ideas since they can refer to different aspects of the human being.

That is, a person may have, for example, high self-esteem in terms of intellectual abilities - I am very clever in mathematics - but low self-esteem in other areas, for example, "I am very clumsy in sports."

### 1. Bright shining self-esteem

People with highly inflated self-esteem are characterized by being very confident in their abilities. In this way, they can make decisions, take risks, and face tasks with a high expectation of success because they see themselves positively.

As our bright self-esteem increases, we will feel better prepared, with greater capacity and disposition to carry out various activities; we will have tremendous enthusiasm and desire to share with others.

### 2. Dull less intense self-esteem

People with self-esteem lacking brightness can feel insecure, dissatisfied, and sensitive to criticism. Another characteristic of people with low self-esteem can be the difficulty of being assertive, or claiming their rights adequately.

Dull shining self-esteem can come from various reasons, such as the appreciation we make of ourselves, the opinion we have of our personality, and our beliefs.

In the same way, they can sometimes try to please others to receive positive reinforcement and, in this way, increase their self-esteem.

Complete the following entry from the Glow Up and Sparkle journal:

When I look in the mirror, I see...


## Characteristics of less intense self-esteem

Typically, a person with dull less intense self-esteem:

• Is extremely critical of herself

• Minimize or ignore their positive qualities.

• Judges herself as inferior to her peers.

• Say things like "stupid," "fat," "ugly," or "unlovable" to describe yourself.

• Having constant negative, critical, and self-blaming debates with themselves (this is referred to as "self-talk").

• She assumes that luck plays an important role in all she achievements and does not take credit for them.

• Blames themselves when things go wrong instead of considering other things over which they have no control, such as the actions of other people or other forces.

• If anyone praises you, don't trust them.

Dull self-esteem and quality of life.

Low self-esteem can reduce a person's quality of life in many different ways, including:

• Negative emotions: chronic self-criticism can lead to feelings of sadness, depression, anxiety, frustration, shame, or guilt.

• Relationship problems: for example, they can tolerate all kinds of irrational behavior from their partners because they believe that love and friendship must be earned, that they cannot be loved or are not kind. An individual with low self-esteem, on the other hand, can become enraged and bully others.

• Fear of trying: the person may doubt her abilities or her worth and avoid challenges.

• Perfectionism: a person can strive and become an achiever to "atone for" what she sees as her inferiority.

• Fear of being judged negatively: they may avoid activities involving other people, such as sports or social gatherings, because they are afraid of being judged negatively. The person feels self-conscious and stressed with others and constantly looks for "signs" that people do not like them.

• Low resilience: a person with low self-esteem has difficulty coping with a challenging event in life because she already believes that she is "desperate."

• Lack of self-care: the person may worry so little that she neglects or abuses herself, for example, she drinks too much alcohol.

• Self-injurious behaviors: low self-esteem puts the person at greater risk of self-harm, for example, eating disorder, drug abuse or suicide

## Causes of a less intense self-esteem

## Some of the many causes of low self-esteem can include:

• Unhappy childhood in which parents (or other important people, such as teachers) were extremely critical

• Lack of confidence as a result of poor academic performance in school.

• Ongoing stressful life event, such as a relationship breakdown or financial problems

• Abuse from a partner, parent, or caregiver (for example, being in an abusive relationship).

• A persistent medical condition, such as chronic pain, a severe illness, or a physical disability

• Anxiety disorders or depression are examples of mental illnesses.

Get support from a professional therapist or counselor, if you're having severe problems with your self-esteem.

Chronic issues can be discouraging and lead to low self-esteem. Get professional help if you're having trouble with your relationship, anxiety, or finances.

Complete the following entry from the Glow Up and Sparkle journal:

Somethings that make me (beautiful) Be You T Full are...

# Promotion of self-esteem

Self-esteem is strongly related to how you see and react to things that happen in your life. Suggestions for building self-esteem include:

• Talk to yourself in a positive way: treat yourself as you would your best friend. Be understanding, kind, and understanding.

• Refute negative "self-talk": If you judge yourself, take a step back and search for empirical proof that the critique is valid. (If you feel like you can't be objective, ask a trusted friend for their opinion.) You will find that most of your negative self-talk is unfounded.

• Don't compare yourself to others: recognize that we are all different and that each human life has value in its own right. Make a conscious effort to embrace yourself as you are, flaws and all.

• Acknowledge the positive: For example, don't ignore compliments, dismiss their accomplishments as "bad luck," or ignore their positive traits.

• Appreciate your special qualities: remember your good points every day. (If you're having trouble thinking of anything positive to say about yourself, enlist the help of a trusted friend.)

• Forget the past: focus on living in the here and now rather than reliving old hurts and disappointments.

• Give yourself a positive message every day: Buy a set of "inspirational cards" and start reading a new card each day and carry the message of the card with you all day.

• Stop worrying: "worrying" is simply worrying about the future. Accept that you cannot see or change the future and try to keep your thoughts in the here and now.

• Have fun - Schedule enjoyable events and activities for each week.

• Exercise: It's a great brain boost for all kinds of things, but especially for fighting depression and helping you feel good. Goals should be step-by-step, like starting with a walk around the block once a day, signing up for a local gym class, or going swimming.

• Be assertive: Be frank and truthful in communicating your desires, wishes, thoughts, values, and views to others.

• Practice the above tips every day: It takes effort and vigilance to replace unhelpful thoughts and behaviors with healthier versions. Give yourself time to establish new habits. Keep a journal or journal to record your progress. Use the Glow Up and Sparkle journal as well.

# 5 tips for a glowing self-esteem:

If you want to strengthen your self-esteem, you have to keep one thing in mind: this depends solely on you. Remember that self-esteem is, etymologically speaking, the "esteem" you have for yourself ("self"). Therefore, you have to start trying to better the relationship with yourself to be more comfortable with who you are.

But we know that this path is not always easy. Therefore, here are 5 tips for you to learn how to increase self-esteem in women and that you can start feeling better right away.

**1.** You are you

One of the first mottos that you have to put in your mind is that you are you. And, therefore, you have to learn to love and respect      that person that you are inside and outside. Stop comparing yourself to others and focus your attention on yourself. If there is something you do not like, change it. If you feel jealous of others' lives, analyze where they come from and what you can do to overcome them. You must stop placing your focus on the outside and begin to focus it on yourself. There is the first step.

**2.** Cultivate your concerns and your passion
To strengthen self-esteem in women, it is important that you

like yourself and that you like the life you lead. Many times, we let ourselves get carried away by the wheel of routine, and we end up living in an automated way: going to work, doing housework, making food ... But, in the end, all day (or all week) We haven't spent a single minute on ourselves. And that cannot be. You must begin to enjoy time in your own company to be comfortable with yourself. Go to the gym, read for a while, get a massage, listen to music ... Do whatever you want but do it!

**3.** The priority is you

Lack of self-esteem can come because you always put yourself last. This is something widespread in the case of women, especially when they are mothers. The children and the partner become the priority, and they are in the queue. This is a severe mistake. That you are a mother or a woman does not mean that you stop being you. So, remember your position in your life, put yourself first, and consider your tastes, opinions, and desires. If you start to conquer your place in your life, you will begin to feel better about yourself and enjoy greater self-esteem.

**4.** Cultivate an optimistic view of yourself

To improve your self-esteem, you must stop being your worst judge. Self-criticism is always pleasing when it is constructive. Most of the time, if we have low self-esteem, the most common is that self-destructive opinions are created that become original works that we put ourselves on. Therefore, it is essential that you begin to change your inner speech and that, instead of crushing yourself so much for everything that you do not do well, you begin to value everything positive in you.

**5.** Learn to forgive yourself: nobody is

A key aspect of strengthening self-esteem in women is that you keep in mind that nobody is perfect. And, of course, neither are you. Besides, if you admire someone around you, you have to bear in mind that it is most likely that this person is not completely comfortable with herself. We live in a society with a very high level of self-demand, which is even more evident among women. Therefore, we recommend that you relax and forgive yourself for everything that you have gone through, put up with, or are lacking in. Accepting imperfections and hugging you for them is a very healthy thing that you have to do.

# 3 Exercises to brighten self-esteem

To strengthen self-esteem, you can do some exercises that will help you realize your worth and begin to improve the relationship you have with yourself. Often, when we have low levels of self-esteem, we do not value ourselves, which can happen because we do not take time to know ourselves or know who we are or what we want. We must stop for a moment and reconcile with ourselves because, after all, we are the only person who, for sure, is with us all our lives.

Exercise 1: List your strengths

If you have low self-esteem, you are likely very aware of what your faults and defects. But do you remember all the good things you possess? You must take time to remember what is positive in you and that, little by little, the balance is balanced. You are not        perfect, but you are not imperfect either, so the first exercise to raise self-esteem that we propose is to create a list of your strengths.

For this reason, I recommend you get a pen and paper and do the following:

Write the compliments that people who love you tell you (if you are good, polite, nice, generous, etc.)

Write the virtues that you consider you have

Write down everything you are proud of, all the achievements, or goals you have accomplished throughout your life.

Now, put this list on the fridge, on the mirror, or in your

closet to always remember that, even if you don't see it sometimes, you are also an extraordinary person.

## Exercise 2: Pamper Yourself

We spend a large part of our lives planning goals and objectives that we want to achieve. But when we finally get them done, we spend very little time enjoying this self-achievement. And this is a big mistake. We have to dedicate the same time to the enjoyment of what has been achieved and the work to achieve it. Therefore, I recommend that you give yourself a gift when you fulfil any of your purposes. Recognize your effort and reward yourself. When I completed my doctorates degree, I never celebrated. One of my sons completed his doctorates degree the same time. Our graduate was literally the same day. I attended his graduation and not mine. We had two celebrations for him but I never celebrated me. I had many obstacles that take place during the completion of this degree and I truly regret not celebrating me. The good thing is that it's never too late to celebrate.

Also, I recommend that you do not forget to take care of yourself every day. Living in the present is essential to be able to enjoy a much more fulfilling and satisfying life. Therefore, do not leave happiness for tomorrow: have it today. To do this, each day you should dedicate a little time to yourself. It doesnot have to be something exaggerated but, simply, give yourself a daily gift to take care of yourself and love yourself: a chocolate bar,a relaxing bath, a bike ride, meditate, listen to that musical group that you like so much ...

## Exercise 3: Positive Affirmations

To strengthen self-esteem in women, I recommend that you try to change your harmful speech. And for this, a good way is to repeat a series of positive "mantras" that can help you transform your prism. Although it may seem silly, the truth is that reminding yourself of positive things daily is a perfect practice to control your mind and avoid the appearance of negative thoughts.

**Positive Affirmations may include:**

I'm more than enough.

I love life.

I am beautiful on the inside and outside.

I am the architect of my life.

My body is healthy.

My relationship is becoming stronger.

I am becoming stronger in my relationship.

Happiness is a choice.

I recognize my worth.

Do this exercise to raise your self-esteem, I recommend looking in the mirror and drawing a smile. You must begin to make peace with yourself and begin to love and respect yourself every day. Once you are creating this atmosphere, it is time to start talking to yourself, giving yourself positive messages such as the following:

- I can deal with everything that I propose
- I'm not perfect, and nothing happens
- I forgive myself for my defects, and I love myself

for myvirtues
- My happiness depends only on me
- I'm going to get everything that I set my mind to
- You are beautiful, intelligent, strong, and friendly
- I respect and take care of myself
- I trust myself, and I love myself

## Other ways to a sparkling self-esteem include:

- • Discuss your low self-esteem with a trusted friend or loved one.

- • Explore the Better Health channel for more information.

- • Consult your physician for information, advice, and possible referral.

- • Read books on personal development.

- • Take a personal development course.

- • Discuss your problems and get advice from a trained therapist.

Complete the following entry from the Glow Up and Sparkle journal:

I am thankful for......

# TECHNIQUES TO GLOW UP YOURSELF CONFIDENCE

People with high levels of confidence have both (a) high self-efficacy and (b) little fear of failure. Self-efficacy is one's belief in one's ability to succeed and involves a positive evaluation of one's abilities. The low fear of failure is related to the propensity to leave the comfort zone. Self-confidence building techniques address self-efficacy, fear of failure, or both.

**Challenging self-limited beliefs**

**There are three steps to challenging your self-limiting beliefs and reconfiguring your inner narrative:**

1. Identify your self-limiting beliefs. Some of you may already be aware of your inner doubts and fears. Some of you may need to spend some time digging deeper to identify the thoughts that are preventing you from taking action. A good way to identify your self-limiting beliefs is to monitor your emotional triggers. If there are particular situations that make you feel anxious or scared, take some time to reflect on what beliefs are driving those emotions. Being aware of your inner narrative during the course of a day can help you articulate your self-limiting beliefs. See if you minimize your achievements and when or if you attribute your successes to others or to luck. Also observe any comparisons you make of yourself with others. Comparisons are often skewed: we notice the external successes of others, but we do not see their internal struggles, insecurities and limitations. We focus on our own imperfections and do not recognize our achievements.

2. Challenge your self-limiting beliefs. Once you've identified your self-limiting beliefs, whether in the form of self-doubt, downplaying your accomplishments, or negatively comparing yourself to others, we must challenge those beliefs by looking for contradicting evidence. Find the counterargument to your self-limiting belief. If you find this difficult to do, try to distance yourself from your self-limiting belief by imagining that you are training a friend on how to challenge your self-limiting belief. How would you dissuade them from that negative self-talk and convince them otherwise? Then put the advice into practice in your own case.

3. Alter the storyline. The third stage entails replacing your self-limiting beliefs with a more logical, realistic, and positive tale.

**Own your achievements**

Studies show that women tend to give credit to circumstances or other people for their successes. When you attribute your successes to factors outside of you, it undermines confidence.

Why do women do this? Some argue that women may not own their achievements for fear of contravening female roles by being perceived as immodest, competitive, or boastful. From an early age, girls learn to downplay their accomplishments as a way to build relationships with other girls.

Practice recognizing your skills by charting "highlights" from your academic, professional, and personal life. Think about the internal resources and capabilities that supported each achievement and write them down. When in doubt, check your chart of achievements.

**Positive visualization**

Another proven technique for building confidence and improving performance is positive visualization. The neurons in our brain, those electrically excitable cells that relay information, perceive the images as equal to a real-life action, according to research using brain imaging. When we envision a movement, the brain sends an impulse to our neurons telling them to "perform" the movement. This creates a new neural pathway, groups of cells in our brain that work together to create memories or learned behaviors, which prepares our body to act in a manner consistent with what we imagine. All of this occurs without actually engaging in physical activity, but a similar result is achieved. We're fired up and ready to go after our target.

In positive psychology, positive visualization involves imagining your best possible self. Imagining your best possible self helps you clarify your end goals. With a well-defined idea of what you want to achieve, you are in a better position to identify the concrete steps you need to realize your best possible self.

**Growth mindset**

Since fear of failure can hold women back, it is important that women have strategies and tools to contain and cope with failure.

The theory of mindset, supported by research by Stanford University researcher Carol Dweck, offers people a cognitive framework for thinking about failure that can be empowering rather than limiting. Dweck's studies show that the key to success is not ability per se, but whether an individual believes that her abilities are fixed (fixed mindset) or malleable (growth mindset). People with a fixed mindset perceive each performance as a measure of their abilities, while people with a growth mindset perceive performance as a tool to develop their skills. People with a fixed mentality avoid circumstances that could reveal their flaws. This prevents these people from leaving their comfort zone and taking the risks necessary to develop new skills. Growth-minded individuals, on the other hand, view every opportunity as a learning opportunity that can bring them closer to achieving their goals.

Growth mindsets can be created, according to Dweck's study, and cultivating a growth mindset has dramatic positive effects on success. Similar to developing favorable attributions of failure (above) To change one's mindset from a fixed to a growth mindset, one must pay close attention to one's internal discourse and actively replace fixed mindset beliefs with more positive growth mindset beliefs.

## 1. Stop comparing yourself to others

We've been socialized to be competitive, so it's easy to compare ourselves to others. But it can be dangerous. It just doesn't make sense to compare yourself to anyone else on the planet because there is only one. Rather, focus on yourself and your journey. The energy shift, by itself, will help you feel free.

## 2. Don't be concerned with what other people think.

Similarly, don't be concerned about what society thinks or expects of you. You can't make everyone happy so this is a waste of time and will only set you back on your journey to be the best you.

## 3. Allow yourself to make mistakes

"No one is perfect; we all make mistakes," we are told repeatedly from a young age. However, when you grow older, you'll feel more pressure to never fail. Cut yourself some slack! Make mistakes so you can change and learn from them. Accept your history. You're still shifting and evolving from who you were to who you are now to who you will be in the future.

So, ignore the voice in your head that tells you that you have to be fine. Make mistakes, a lot of them! The lessons you will get are priceless.

## 4. Keep in mind that your worth is not determined by your physical appearance.

This is essential! So many things in the world are attempting to divert your attention away from this life-changing reality. Your own internalized misogyny will reinforce your feelings of inadequacy. You are important because of who you are, not because of what you look like.

So, use what makes you feel good. Whether it's a lot or a little, wear whatever makes you feel safe, comfortable, and happy.

## 5. Don't be afraid to let toxic people go

Not everyone takes responsibility for the energy they put out to the world. If there is someone who is bringing toxicity into your life and is not taking responsibility for it, that could mean that you should stay away from them. Don't be afraid to do this. It is liberating and important, even though it can be painful.

Remember: protect your energy. It is not rude or wrong to walk away from situations or the company of people that are wearing you out.

## 6. Process your fears

Like erring, feeling fear is natural and human. Don't reject your fears, understand them. This beneficial exercise will significantly improve your mental health. Questioning and analyzing your fears will help you gain insight and uncover the issues that were causing you anxiety in the first place. As a result, some, if not all, of your anxiety might be relieved.

## 7. Have faith in your ability to make sound choices for yourself.

Too often we doubt ourselves and our ability to do the right thing, when most of the time we know in our hearts what is best. Remember that your feelings are valid. You are not losing touch with reality. You know yourself better than anyone, so be your best advocate.

## 8. Take advantage of all the opportunities that life presents or create your own.

The next big step in your life will never be perfectly timed. The settings may not be ideal, but that shouldn't stop you from achieving your goals and dreams. Instead, seize the moment because you may never come back.

## 9. Put yourself first

Don't feel bad about doing this. Women especially can get used to putting others first. Although there is a time and place for this, it should not be a habit that costs you your mental or emotional well-being.

Find the time to unzip. Without decompressing and reloading, it can take a lot of effort. Whether it's spending the day in bed or outside in nature, find what helps you relax and take time for it.

## 10. Feel the pain and joy to the fullest extent possible.

Allow yourself to truly experience everything. Lean into your suffering, revel in your joy, and don't be afraid to express yourself. Pain and joy, like fear, are emotions that can help you better understand yourself and know that you are not your feelings.

## 11. Exercise boldness in public

Get in the habit of speaking your mind in a respectful manner. Boldness is a muscle that gets stronger with use. Don't wait for permission to sit at the table. Join the conversation. Contribute your thoughts. Take action and know that your voice is as important as anyone else's.

## 12. See the beauty in simple things.

Try to notice at least one small, beautiful thing around you every day. Make a note of it and thank it. Gratitude doesn't just give your perspective, it's essential to help you find joy.

## 13. Be kind to yourself

The world is full of harsh and critical words. Don't add yours to the mix. Speak kindly to yourself and don't call yourself bad things. Celebrate yourself. You have come so far and you have grown a lot. Don't forget to celebrate yourself, and not just on your birthday!

## 14. Put off

Consider how far you've come and how you've lived, even if you don't feel especially strong. You are alive and strong beyond your comprehension right now. And be patient with yourself. Self-love may not happen overnight. But in time, it will settle in your heart.

Yes, you may have a hard time, but you will remember these moments and see how they were stepping stones on your journey to being the best of you.

# Benefits to glowing your self-confidence

These benefits are deeper and broader than most people realize. Increasing your self-confidence will benefit you professionally, whether you are a leader, manager, sales representative, or individual contributor. It will support you personally by assisting you in leading your family and also making you feel and appear sexier to others. Yes, confidence is sexy!

## Here are the 12 benefits of increased self-confidence:

**1. Be your best under stress.** Athletes, singers, and actors will testify to the value of having a high degree of self-assurance. When you're optimistic, you're more likely to reach your full potential and want to give it your all when the stakes are highest, such as when you're under pressure.

**2.Influence other people.** Self-assured people have an easier time influencing others. This comes in handy when pitching an idea or a product, as well as when bargaining at work or at home.

**3. Have a strong corporate and leadership presence.** In terms of leadership and executive presence, self-assurance is crucial. How you think, behave (including how you hold yourself), and use your voice all contribute to your presence.

**4. Exude a more positive attitude.** When you are secure in yourself, you believe you have a significant and meaningful role to play in the world, which gives you a positive outlook.

**5. Feeling valued.** When you're confident in yourself, you know what you're good at and that you're valuable.

**6. Climbing to the top.** Looking for a promotion? The more self-assured you are, the more likely you are to advance in your career.

**7. Be sexier.** Did you know that confidence is sexy?

**8. Reduce negative thoughts.** Increased self-confidence allows you to experience freedom from self-doubt and negative thoughts about yourself.

**9. Experience more courage and less anxiety.** Greater confidence makes you more willing to take smart risks and better able to step out of your comfort zone.

**10. Have greater freedom from social anxiety.** Feeling more comfortable being yourself reduces worry about what others may think of you. How liberating!

**11. Get energy and motivation to act.** Confidence provides you with the motivation to act and accomplish your personal and professional goals. The more motivated and energetic you are, the more likely you are to take immediate action.

**12. Be happier.** People who are self-assured are happier and more content with their lives than those who are not.

# Habits of a confident woman

When you hear "confident woman," most people will automatically have an image of someone who resonates in their mind. This person is easily noticed, portrays success and radiates happiness. They are the perfect image of "confidence."

But what do these people have that gives them confidence? As with most characteristics, there are some behaviors of positive women that you can incorporate into your life to boost your esteem and, as a result, your happiness.

The 11 habits of a self-assured woman are mentioned below. You don't need to have all of them to be confident, but it would be very difficult to find a confident woman who doesn't have some of these for sure.

## 1 - She questions the "norm"

You will seldom find a confident woman who goes with the flow, never questioning what she is told, what the "norm" is, and simply being remarkably average.

I am not talking about women who argue all the points, or even women who find Zen in allowing life to unfold in "flow", but even more about those who never question the "why".

Why are you doing what you are doing? Is that because this is how it's always been done? Is there a better way?

She's not afraid to say "actually, no, that doesn't work for me, let's try it this way." Even beyond that, she's not afraid to say "that didn't really work, let's try something different again."

## 2 - She reserves the word "Yes" for when she really says it

We all know that person (maybe even you) who says yes to everything!! She doesn't want to disappoint anyone. But in doing so, she always ends up doing it for others and not for herself.

Sounds familiar?

"No" is a difficult word for many people to say. That is because it is direct and definitive. A "no" ends a conversation and is a strong term that can be hurtful if used incorrectly.

A confident woman knows that saying "no" to others often means that she is saying "yes" to herself.

And when you say "yes" to others, you have to be serious. Because it usually means that you will give up something for yourself (time, energy) and when you say yes, you don't mean it and you mean it. That's why a "yes" from a confident woman means so much.

**3 - She uses positive words in her conversations**

One of my business mentors once told me how vital our words are. Her example had to do with simple words that we use in our daily conversations.

Instead of saying "don't forget", he explained that instead she said "please remember". We are much more likely to respond to positive than negative words.

A confident woman uses positive words in her conversations to edify herself and others. She doesn't have to put other people down to feel good about herself.

You will be motivated after a talk with a confident woman.

**4 - Has clear goals and action plans to achieve them**

A confident woman understands that while goals are important, they mean nothing unless she has a plan of action to achieve them.

She's fine to sit here and say "my goal is to make enough money so I can quit my job," and that's fantastic. But unless she has a plan in place for how she's going to achieve it, her goal is nothing more than a dream.

Goals, action plans, and follow-up are areas that a confident woman understands and uses well.

She uses planner or journal to help her create and track her goals:

**5 - She knows that confidence is much more than appearance, but she knows the benefits of "her power team"**

Everyone has at least one outfit or piece of clothing that helps them feel confident, powerful, and like they can conquer the world. Her power teams.

And while we know that confidence is about much more than looks, we also understand that any little confidence boost we can get, even if it comes from a perfectly fitted pair of pants and amazing heels, it's worth it.

**6 - She shows confident body language**

Imagine Wonder Woman ... with only more clothes on and less wind machine moving her hair.

However, there is a lot of psychology behind the advantages of the power pose, and a confident woman knows how to use it to her advantage. Even when she doesn't feel very confident that day, she knows that she can fake it until she does it with a pose of power.

Also, she will rarely see her slumped or cowering in the crowd. A confident woman stands upright, she looks people in the eye when she talks to them and smiles, because she believes in herself.

## 7 - You have a good understanding of your own personality, including your strengths and weaknesses

Understanding yourself can be crucial to your success. A confident woman is aware of her own strengths and limitations and knows how to exploit them.

She may be able to better convey her message when she speaks, but it really is hard for him to write her thoughts. Simple solution: she records what she wants to say and ask a transcriber to write it for you.

You may know that she is much more patient around 10 am when she has had time to drink her coffee, answer emails, and write her to-do list for the day. Fantastic: you know she shouldn't book any meetings until after that time.

## 8 – She creates her own success without feeling the need to bring down others

A confident woman would never say, "Well, I did better than you," because she understands that her own success is unrelated to the shortcomings of others.

She her successes are hers; she works hard to achieve them and she understands that the other successes are the same.

The comparison is not a trap that she falls into (too often) and she is happy to help someone celebrate her own success, even if she has not yet achieved hers.

## 9 - She focuses on the positive and leaves negative behaviors (and people) behind

Being around a confident woman is like getting a massive boost of positivity in your day. She has little time for the world's Negative Nellies and eliminates them from her life.

She has this amazing ability to see the bright side of any situation, and she leaves you feeling motivated.

She sure has her bad days, everyone does. She can't be 100 percent optimistic all of the time because it would be unthinkable. She, on the other hand, tries to see the good in the world and surrounds herself with positive people and stuff.

10 - She understands the importance of personal care

A confident woman knows that the first person she must take care of is herself. Because if she can't take care of herself, then she can't take care of anyone else.

She schedules regular self-care activities, even if it means getting up a half hour early so you can sit down and drink her coffee while she's still warm.

Personal care is the backbone of success in every way. A self-assured woman understands that pushing herself to the limit to achieve success is pointless because she is not sustainable.

While she may not like her, she also agrees to speak up when she needs help and when she needs to take time out.

**11 - She steps out of her comfort zone**

Whether you're an extrovert, an introvert, or somewhere in between, stepping out of your comfort zone can be difficult. But a confident woman knows that she has never accomplished anything great within her comfort zone.

While it may take her some time, and some major efforts to make this happen, a confident woman is still fine if she steps out of her comfort zone from time to time. In fact, she encourages it.

She understands that the only way she can develop is to push her limits, and she is confident in her ability to do so.

How does your confidence weigh at the moment? Are there areas you want to work on to increase her confidence?

We are not always 100% sure all the time, but if we do at least some of these things, most of the time, we will be moving towards a more confident and successful woman.

# Ways to concentrate on your personal development as a woman

Personally, I am so caught up in everything I have to do that sometimes I miss opportunities to grow. Sometimes it's because I completely pass them on in my effort to complete my to-do list and other times. I'm honestly too tired to push myself (am I the only one collapsing on the couch with some Netflix after work?).

Growth looks different for every woman because we are all in completely different stages and places in our lives, but here are some things that have really helped me grow as a woman.

**Spend time with other women.**

The significance of this one cannot be overstated. I may seem to feel diminished by other women in my darkest and most vulnerable areas, and it wasn't until college that I realized how much I was missing. I began investing in my female friendships, and I now have a wonderful tribe of women who I admire and respect, and who continually encourage and challenge me to be the best version of myself. Screenwriters, moms, educators, counselors, nurses, social workers, and the list goes on and are they among my closest friends. Even though some of them live long distances, we do our best to keep in touch and it's like no time has passed when we catch up. I cannot imagine my life without them, and all the seasons of life for which they have accompanied me, with their prayers, their laughter and their encouragement.

**Take ballroom dancing lessons.**

Okay, this may sound crazy to some of you ladies, but listen to me. I've spent much of my young adult life trying to blend in, to hide, to stay out of the spotlight. I didn't even feel particularly elegant, strong, or beautiful. So, I chose something that interested me and that I felt embodied everything that was not, everything that could not be, and I did. I was amazed at how difficult it was for me to put myself in a position that felt so vulnerable. What if my instructors see me make mistakes? What if I looked ridiculous? What if I never got better? For me, showing up every week for my lesson took Wonder Woman's strength, but doing it over and over again I found that I liked seeing a new side of myself. I even did a dance recital, and although I was incredibly nervous, I was very proud that I had overcome my fear and developed a new sense of confidence.

**Spend time with books.**

I love to sit and read, but I find less and less time to sit and read a physical book. I still do, but it's getting harder and harder to find a time for it these days. For the rest of you ladies in the same boat,

I highly recommend checking out Audible. It's perfect for listening while cleaning, commuting, relaxing on the beach, etc. There is a $ 15 monthly fee to use the app after your free trial, but you get a free credit for any audiobook every month. with option to buy more. Most of the book's cost between $ 15 and $ 20 anyway, so it's a good investment from my perspective.

 In fact, I've heard it twice (and will probably do it again) and would definitely recommend it to any woman who wants to be challenged and overcome insecurity.

**Listen to podcasts.**

Like listening to Audible to spruce up your book, if you're looking for shorter pieces to commit to (think TV episodes vs. a full movie), there are always podcasts. Whether you're looking for educational content, entertainment, sermons, or just something generally encouraging, podcasts can be downloaded or streamed to your phone.

**Go traveling.**

It is a true saying that wherever you go, there you are. You won't magically become a different person overnight by changing locations, but it is difficult to remain unchanged when exposed to new places. With every place you visit, whether it's a new coffee shop in town or a whole new continent, you'll meet new people, try new foods, hear new sounds and music, and see something you haven't seen before. Going to new places means experiencing things differently - laying the foundation for the opportunity to develop a new perspective.

**Volunteer.**

This is a really great and easy way to help her grow as a woman. There are so many great organizations working for each and every cause, you can imagine. Taking time to give back to others and a chance to work toward a common goal can create a sense of purpose and balance in our otherwise hectic schedules.

I believe that sometimes we make personal growth distant and unattainable when often all we really need to do is intentionally seize our opportunities. Taking a cooking class can seem more time consuming than listening to a podcast on the way to work, but the goals are the same. Living a life of courage and grace means operating with intention at all opportunities.

# How to make your self-confidence glow

*Everyone can do things to gain more security. Here are a few tips to try:*

1. **Capable", retrain it to say: "I can", "I am capable".** You could also speak to yourself, "I know I can learn (or build an attitude of mental confidence. When your inner voice says: "I cannot" or "I am not do) this if I give my full attention."
2. **Be kind to yourself when comparing yourself to others**. It is usual for us to compare ourselves with other people. It is a way of understanding ourselves and developing those qualities that we admire. But if comparisons often leave you feeling bad about yourself, this is a sign that you need to do something to improve your self-confidence and self-esteem.
3. **Get rid of doubts about yourself.** When we still doubt our abilities, we feel inferior, invalid, unworthy, or unprepared. This can make us avoid people and situations that we might enjoy,

which could help us grow.

4. **Challenge yourself to do something outdoor in your usual comfort zone.** Choose something that you would like to do if you had more confidence in yourself. Give yourself a push and do it. Once you've done it, choose something else, give it a try, and keep repeating this same process. Your self-confidence will grow with each new step you take forward.

5. **Recognize your talent and let it shine.** They teach us to work hard to improve our weak points. Sometimes it is important, like when we get poor grades in school and realize that we have to try harder. Don't let working on your weaknesses prevent you from improving even more what you already do well.

6. **Show yourself as you are.** Let others see you and love you for who you are, with your mistakes, your insecurities, and everything else. It is easier to overcome insecurity when we do not feel that we should hide it. Assume and accept your quirks instead of trying to be like someone else or acting in a way that is not yours.

7. **It takes courage and self-confidence to be authentic.** But the more authentic we are, the more confident we will become. Confidence in ourselves increases our self-esteem.

# GLOW UP TO SELF- LOVE

Self-love is the acceptance, respect, perceptions, value, positive thoughts and considerations that we have towards ourselves, and those around us can appreciate that.

Self-love depends on our will to love ourselves, not on those around us or on the situations or contexts we do not develop.

Self-love reflects what the relationship is like and the feelings we have for ourselves, physique, personality, character, attitudes and behaviors.

In general, it is said that before loving another person, we must first love ourselves to know how to value ourselves, recognize that we deserve good and beautiful things throughout life and that we are worthy of loving and being loved.

Happiness is the main goal of self-love, being happy to accept ourselves as we are without letting external people outside our family and circle of loved ones intervene.

Family and education are fundamental bases to build and strengthen self-love.

At home, the parents and loved ones have the responsibility to strengthen, from an early age, confidence in ourselves and understand how important it is to accept ourselves as we are and know how to recognize our strengths and weaknesses.

People who feel self-love are characterized by being friendly, respectful, loving, independent. They cherish their personal growth, their state of health, their training and give their best in all the activities they develop.

Over the centuries, women and their desires have been relegated to patriarchal society. Women thought that being a "good mother and wife" was loving herself. They felt that enduring abuse, enduring in silence, satisfying others... meant loving herself.

Fortunately, times are changing little by little. In reality, there is still   a long way to go towards equality between women and men.  However, each woman brings change personally by loving herself by prioritizing her desires and dreams.

For female empowerment, these habits of self-love can be very positive. Among them is allowing yourself to dream, allowing yourself to fulfil those dreams, having a natural and healthy body, allowing yourself to go out or stay. In short, learn to dive into your desires and feelings, to know what is or is not good for each one.

My mother never told me about self-love but she would always say "love yourself first". In other words, put yourself first.   It's called self-care.  While traveling on the airplane, we are informed by the flight attendant to give yourself oxygen first so that you will be able to give others oxygen

## Some characteristics of self-love are:

- ○ You love yourself; you  respect yourself, and you value yourself,
- ○ You have high self-esteem,
- ○ You know who you are and what you want
- ○ You feel happy and abundant
- ○ You accept yourself as you are
- ○ You have a nice relationship with your physical body,
- ○ You feel worthy of loving and of being loved,
- ○ You feel worthy
- ○ You have confidence in yourself
- ○ You do your best.

# Habits That Destroy Your Self-Love

1.  Disqualifying yourself

When you're the one who talks bad about yourself, you're not doing yourself any favors. It is not a sign of recognition of your mistakes. It is a mechanism that reveals a kind of autosuggestion.

Disqualifying yourself is being trapped in those criticisms of the past and that you now use so as not to forget that you have no right to look at yourself in another way

But you are much more than everything they told you. You have many virtues and potentials to discover; you have to start accepting and loving yourself to see yourself beyond others' eyes.

**2.** Give absolute credit to what others say

You may feel that others "know more," or "understand better," or "have more authority" to say or do. You do not stop to evaluate if what others say or do is correct; it is enough for you that they are the ones who say or do.

If you stop to think for a bit, you may find that this is not the case.    Always try to connect with your true perception and value what you see.

### 3. Victimize you

In the face of difficulties, your response may be to feel sorry for yourself. You perceive yourself as a helpless child who must resign herself to negative situations without doing anything about it.

You have not discovered that you have the resources to face    adverse situations. That the important thing is not how bad it happens, but how we receive it and its course. If you stopped complaining about yourself and started thinking about solutions, you would discover that even the worst moments are also great opportunities.

### 4. Demand more of you than the bill

Those who have little self-esteem tend to see life in terms of ideal    models. It is difficult for her to set modest goals and assess the achievements. She always thinks that she must achieve more and that what she has achieved may not be important. It is a cold trap to always be in debt to yourself.

Don't be afraid to congratulate yourself on every step you take. Big goals are built with little links.

If you do not have self-love, nothing you do will be enough or valuable. Your successes will be worth nothing compared to the achievements of others. But make no mistake, if you do not start by valuing yourself, it will not be easy for others. How are you going to appreciate yourself if you cannot applaud yourself when you move forward?

To achieve the goal of a full and happy life, it can be key to integrate these habits of self-love in the course of a day.

## 1. Self-love habits: listening to yourself

Follow your wishes to achieve the goals you set for yourself as a woman.

It seems obvious, but women are always conditioned by the social opinion that weighs on them. Most cultures have viewed women as a commodity or as a domestic worker. The raising of one's children or the children of others were female duties.

It has not been easy to conquer rights, and in many countries, women are still deprived of them. However, in the West, you can choose lifestyles with relative freedom. Relative, because if a woman does not want children or a husband, she will be judged by a society sector, even by her own family.

For all these reasons, listening to one's desire is the most important of self-love habits. Whether choosing a career, choosing a partner, or choosing a wardrobe, the main thing is to connect with your desire.

## 2. Say yes: total acceptance

The habits of self-love are closely interconnected with each other. Accepting herself with all her flaws is the most beautiful thing a woman can do for herself.

The image of the smiling, submissive, maternal and complacent maiden can now be stamped on old figures and paintings. No one can define what it is to be a woman, nor can one compare one woman to another.

## 3. Allow yourself to be happy

May no one take happiness away from you. Enjoy life as a woman!

Many women remain in unhappy relationships and do not realize that their doors are open to leave.

You have to take that step toward self-esteem, whether in

relations partner, in friendships, at work or in the family.

### 4. This is how it is built

Self-love is built from childhood. When people receive a very authoritarian or very indifferent education, they may not always learn to establish healthy relationships with themselves and with others. They can grow without valuing who they are or what they do.

But this does not mean that someone who has not received a good up bringing cannot learn to love herself.

It's never too late. One of the important tasks of human beings is to learn to love oneself, which is easier when they have received a loving and generous upbringing, during which the child's way of being has been respected.

To start building self-love, it is vital to understand that human beings' value is not given by external factors but by their essence. From there, it is easier to start the path of knowing yourself, of knowing that you are an imperfect being and that, just as you are, you deserve to be loved.

## Phrases to start loving yourself

Positive phrases and affirmations to recover and increase self-love  are a great help and motivation to embark on the journey of loving  yourself.

Here are the ones that resonate the most with me.

1. "To love yourself right now, as you are, is to give yourself  joy. Don't wait until it's too late. If you wait, you lose your joy now. If you love, you live now.

2. "Loving yourself is the beginning of a lifelong romance.

3. "When I loved myself, I started to get rid of everything that was  not healthy: people, situations and anything that pushed me down. At first, my reason called that attitude selfishness. Today it is called... Self-love.

4. "You, as well as anyone else in the entire universe, deserve your love and affection."

5. "Being beautiful means being yourself. You don't need to be accepted by others. You need to accept yourself.

6. "A person cannot be comfortable without her approval.

7. "When I truly loved myself, I understood that in any circumstance, I was in the right place and at the right time. And then, I was able to relax. Today I know that it has a name ... self-esteem.

8. "Self-esteem is a feeling based on feeling capable and loved." Jack Canfield.

9. "If you believe totally in yourself, there will be nothing that is beyond your possibilities." Wayne Dyer.

10. "Self-esteem and self-love are the opposite of fear; the more you love yourself, the less anxiety you will have of doing anything.

11. "Self-esteem is a feeling based on feeling capable and loved.

12. "Love yourself first, and everything else falls into order. You have to love yourself to do anything in this world.

13. "We all know that self-esteem comes from what you think of yourself, not from what others think of you." Gloria Gaynor.

14. "Loving oneself, despising or ignoring others, is presumption and exclusion; loving others, disliking oneself is a lack of self-love.

15. "The learning to love is to appreciate what you see when you look in the mirror."

This is how people who love themselves recognize themselves:

Key points

- Authentic: they don't want to be like anyone else. They want to be who they are.
- Confident: they trust their actions even if they are wrong because they learn.
- Resilient: they always take an opportunity out of the problem.
- They trust others
- Happy and enthusiastic about everything they do

## Conclusion

Self-love, self-esteem, confidence, and dignity are essential to be happy and have the life you want.

Everything, absolutely everything, depends on you. And it is better to start building from within yourself.

Inquire into yourself, explore, dive within yourself. Dedicate yourself to discover who you are and accepting how beautiful you already are.

One day you will realize that you and your lack of love caused everything negative that happened to you in your life, help to make you who you are today. Everything that has happened to me during my life, I use it as a learning experience to help me to be a better me. It is as if it is my motivation to excel and prevail.

Living and vibrating in love will give you everything you need. You will understand that there is no better relationship than the one you have with yourself. If it is based on self-love, then you will have achieved everything. I hope each of you will be able to glow up and sparkle.

www.ingramcontent.com/pod-product-compliance
Lightning Source LLC
Chambersburg PA
CBHW022133280326
41933CB00007B/671